Finding Purpose

Finding Purpose

A Neurosurgeon's Journey of Hope and Healing

Anthony M. Avellino, MD, MBA

A Note to Reader
I have spent many hours researching the information provided in this book. To the best of my knowledge, the information is accurate, and I apologize for any statements that may be inaccurate, and in no way do they reflect upon the institutions or persons cited in this book. I welcome your feedback to my email: findingpurpose37@gmail.com.

Dedication

This book is dedicated to my wife, Jennifer, my daughter, Ashleigh, my son, Michael, and my dog, Parker, who I love and admire greatly. They are the true joys of my life and have given me the courage to inspire others to be their best!

Table of Contents

Foreword

In his book *Finding Purpose: A Neurosurgeon's Journey of Hope and Healing*, my friend and colleague Dr. Anthony M. Avellino makes it clear that we are all fearfully and wonderfully made with loads of potential and the ability to lead good, productive lives. Each of us, however, at some point, makes the decision to control that potential or to be controlled by the events as they unfold in our lives. The key point here is that the direction of our lives can be controlled, and we are not helpless participants on the stage of life.

Stress plays a significant role in all of our lives, whether we realize it or not. I had always heard that neurosurgery was supposed to be highly stressful, and yet, I didn't generally feel stressed. When I retired from neurosurgery, I suddenly realized how stressful it had been. I would wake up in the morning and not be responsible for the lives of critically ill patients, and that was a sensation with which I was unfamiliar. My faith has always played a large role in every aspect of my life, and I gave God the credit for the good as well as the responsibility for the bad. That is perhaps the reason I didn't feel the stress. But when we don't have a good mechanism for dealing with stress, it can become the dominating force in our lives. In this book, Dr. Avellino helps the reader recognize the stressors and deal with them.

Perspective is another very important word when it comes to identifying purpose in one's life. Some years ago, I was asked to lead a team in an attempt to separate twins conjoined at the head in South Africa. The technical aspects of the operation were magnificent, but it turned out that one twin had all the cardiac function, and the other twin had all the kidney function; therefore, they were symbiotic, meaning they couldn't live apart. They could not live together either, because as they grew, they were experiencing progressive heart failure. Needless to say, once they were separated, the one with no heart function died immediately, and the one with no kidney function died days later. I was extremely depressed, asking myself why I needed to get involved in such a horrible failure. A couple of years later, a set of conjoined twins from Zambia were able to be brought to South Africa where we quickly reassembled the team and already had all the equipment and were able to perform the first totally successful complex separation of twins joined at the head. That would not have been possible without the previous failure, which ensured that the team and the equipment were prepared. That kind of perspective made me much more capable of handling both success and failure in future cases.

This book is designed to give the reader insight into the many factors that will determine whether life is a success or failure. Life can be very exciting if the central feature is not oneself and one concentrates on empowering others and improving the general atmosphere in which they exist.

Benjamin S. Carson, Sr., MD

Introduction

Each year, almost 400 physicians die by suicide. Reading that sentence should be enough to give anyone who has dedicated their life to helping and saving others cause for concern.

From the perspective of family, friends, and colleagues, I present as a 54-year-old pediatric neurosurgeon, endurance ultra-runner, husband, father, and friend. Yet, I have battled with the inner demons of depression, obsessive-compulsive tendencies, and stuttering for as long as I can remember.

In becoming a neurosurgeon, I sought to live my life bringing healing to those with neurological disease. After completing my training, I felt a tremendous sense of pride knowing that I was prepared to have a great impact on patients and families in their time of greatest need and hopelessness. I entered and ended each day with the knowledge that I had given my all. I, like many of my colleagues, ignored fatigue and underestimated the accumulated trauma and stress until suddenly,

I became one of the statistics—burned out, depressed, and suicidal. The administrative, clinical, and personal stressors had struck down my physical and mental health.

On September 12, 2009, I attempted suicide. In that particular moment, my resolve was gone, replaced by fear, hopelessness, and a sense of inadequacy. I lacked the skills to respond and was overwhelmed by emotions I had never known. I felt that I was trapped and could not turn to loved ones for support, lest I lose their respect.

I found my way out. My blessing was my family, my resolve, and my mission. I know recovery is possible, because I have recovered through family, friends, and ultra-running. Expressing and acknowledging our insecurities is vital, but it is how we deal with them and find inner peace that is key. Showing compassion and kindness to ourselves and the members of the high functioning teams we lead is vital.

My work in neurosurgery involves the brain health of our patients, and part of maintaining their brain health is taking care of themselves and ourselves while sustaining a work-life balance. We need to raise awareness about physician wellness and remove the stigma and the tendency to keep physician burnout a secret. Burnout can lead to anxiety, depression, suicidal thoughts, marital and family stress, anger issues, addiction, and substance abuse, any of which can lead to dissatisfaction, and ultimately, physicians ending their careers.

Physicians are twice as likely to be dissatisfied with their work-life balance than the average working adult. In 2015, almost 50 percent of physicians reported they were burned out. Medical students' rate of depression is 15–30 percent higher than that of the general public. Physicians are more than twice as likely to take their own lives than the general population. Female physicians are 2.5–4 times as likely to die by suicide than women in other occupations (1).

These are national statistics. We can—and should—do things differently in America. If we recognize and reduce the stressors that lead to burnout, we can create a supportive environment that fosters our own physical and mental well-being. This will allow us to provide the best quality care for our patients.

On June 10, 2016, I decided to speak up and raise awareness of mental health; as often, you hear about someone's depression after they take their life. Part of my everyday living is showing my vulnerability and telling my story to let others know to keep fighting for life and to strive for an effective work-life balance. My efforts over the past four years have been to help colleagues focus on raising awareness of mental health and removing the stigma so that we begin to talk about and develop wellness strategies and overcome the hills of life. I have shared my story countless times with colleagues, medical students, and staff. I do this to destigmatize burnout and let those facing pain in silence know they are not alone. I have also taken the empathy resultant from my pain and turned it into a career focused on healing for the vulnerable.

In June 2018, I was recruited by Michigan State University to help develop a safer and healthier campus, following the sentencing of former USA Gymnastics national team and sports medicine physician Dr. Larry Nassar, who was sent to prison for criminal acts of sexual assault. Under the leadership of Dr. Norman Beauchamp, Executive Vice President for Health Sciences, we are responsible and accountable for the strategic initiatives and programs to increase health, safety, and wellness practices across all Michigan State University's health care services to ensure best practices and exemplary care in a learning and healing environment.

In this memoir, I share my vulnerabilities of stuttering, obsessive-compulsive tendencies, depression, and suicide. We must all listen, learn, and heal with each other to achieve a healthier, peaceful, and purposeful life with optimum performance in mind, body, and spirit. We must remember we are never alone. And we must find hope, even in the darkest moments, for the lessons learned can give us insights on how to bring light to others.

I truly wish I knew 35 years ago what I know today, as I would have lived a more peaceful life. I hope this memoir empowers you to *listen, learn, and heal to find purpose* to be your best and develop an effective work-life balance to achieve a happy, healthy, and extraordinary life.

Part I

Listen (to discover your life's journey)

"If you can dream it, you can do it!"

—WALT DISNEY

MY LIFE JOURNEY

I want to share with you my journey with depression, obsessive-compulsive tendencies, and stuttering, exemplifying how caring people in my life helped me become the person I am today. Born and raised in the Bronx, New York, I attended elementary school at Our Saviour Lutheran School through third grade with predominantly minority students. From this experience, I witnessed the barriers to access and resources. I also learned about cultural diversity and disparities early on, and I formed the opinion that all people are the same regardless of their origin or disability. Subsequently, my family moved to Westchester County, and I attended public schools.

During elementary and high school, I struggled with being imperfect, which to me meant not being good enough. Now I know those were my depressive and obsessive-compulsive tendencies. Managing my stuttering when moving to a new school was challenging. I remember how much fun it was for my classmates to hear me speak and how it was a common pastime for them to get me to talk whenever possible. They would jibe and jeer, asking, "What did you say? Why don't you learn to talk in English?" Their best entertainment was to tease and mock me until I became angry, taunt me when I did, and ridicule me every time. At times, I hated going to school—not because I disliked school, but because I was sure to meet some of my taunting classmates and be humiliated and laughed at because I stuttered. Having reached the school room, I had to face the prospect of failing every time I tried to ask a question or talk to others. However, as I look back at my classmates who helped make my life miserable at times in school, I feel kindness toward them. They made me realize I was "handicapable," which eventually triggered me into reaching out for help.

My dad was an electrician with a high school degree, and my mom never graduated high school. However, they both instilled in me values of being compassionate to others and working hard to achieve my goals. My mom always said to me, "You can do anything that you put your mind to." My parents divorced when I was a teenager, and they both remarried and have been in loving relationships for over 30 years. I was fortunate that my stepfather, Mike Proios, was an incredible and compassionate person who cared deeply about me and always treated me like his own son.

I graduated from Eastchester High School in Eastchester, New York, and was fortunate to attend Cornell University, where I played lightweight football and majored in microbiology and biochemistry. After my sophomore year, I decided to stop playing football, as I sustained a career-ending injury to my left thumb, and I committed to be a physician, my lifelong dream. Giving up football was one of the most difficult life decisions for me, as football provided me with a sense of worth. I didn't know the signs and symptoms of depression, as I always thought it was best to tough it out like I did with playing football, where I continued to play whether tired, sore, or injured.

After graduating from Cornell University, I matriculated at Columbia University College of Physicians & Surgeons, where I had the opportunity to study at a school steeped in tradition for training the next generation of physicians. I was then fortunate to train at the premier University of Washington School of Medicine neurosurgery residency program in Seattle, Washington, under Dr. H. Richard Winn. I completed a pediatric neurosurgery fellowship at Seattle Children's Hospital under the superb direction of Dr. Richard G. Ellenbogen and was recruited to Johns Hopkins University, where I was privileged to be Dr. Ben Carson's partner. I chose a career in pediatric neurosurgery as it allowed me to use my surgical skills while providing the best holistic quality care to children and their families.

As I climbed the ladder to be a neurosurgeon, I was fortunate to have my wife, Jennifer, at my side. We have been married for over 27 years, and she is my best friend, confidante, and soulmate. She continues to be the rock of our family. Her compassion and unconditional love lifts some of the burden when I am working long hours and fatigued.

After my daughter was born, my wife and I had the opportunity to return to the University of Washington, where I had progressive executive and academic leadership and learning opportunities. I obtained my MBA degree and was residency director of the neurosurgery training program, chief of pediatric neurosurgery, inaugural director of the UW Medicine Neurosciences Institute, and chief of neurosurgery.

As a pediatric neurosurgeon, I have had the privilege to experience incredible triumphs and dreadful human suffering with the children and their families that entrusted me with their care. I have seen the power of the human spirit at its best and worst. All these experiences have affected my emotional and physical well-being. Being a physician is an incredible responsibility that brings an enormous amount of joy, happiness, and self-worth. It also has a burden of incredible guilt when explaining the daunting task of moving on when a child's outcome is grim or terminal. The compounding trauma of dealing with uncertainty and not being able to do anything takes its toll over time when one has not developed healthy self-coping mechanisms.

On September 12, 2009, I was in a bad, depressive place with feelings of isolation and loss. While my wife was living her volunteer passion of directing a children's book event, I sat in my car in my garage and hooked up a vacuum hose from my exhaust into my car window and tried to take my life. As I was breathing in carbon monoxide fumes and began to feel sleepy and peaceful, I saw visions of my son, Michael. For some reason, I opened the door, coughed, and stopped. I had hit rock bottom and decided to seek help. I decided that I would call the employee assistance program through my employer and seek counseling help. Over the past 10 years, I have sought help through the employee assistance program twice, and I am grateful and thank God every day that I get to see my wife, son, daughter, and experience the joys of life.

I never told anyone about my suicide attempt except my wife, Jennifer, and my friend, Jake Anderson, who has struggled with depression and substance abuse himself. I was afraid to let anyone know for the fear and stigma of what others would think of me. I was programmed from playing football to never show signs of weakness and to be tough and play through pain. I had obsessive-compulsive tendencies, and I needed to be perfect. I was fearful of losing my job. I went to two Ivy League schools, and I was fearful of losing everything for which I worked so hard. Would my friends, family, and colleagues think I was weak? I was fearful, ashamed, and embarrassed of what others would think.

After my suicide attempt, I committed to develop healthy self-coping skills with compassion, vulnerability, accountability, continuous improvement, and transformational change. I also realized that my life's mission is to help others achieve their optimum performance in mind, body, and spirit so they lead a healthier, peaceful, and purposeful life. No one should ever hit rock bottom as I was.

In August 2014, I was recruited to be the chief executive officer of the OSF HealthCare Illinois Neurological Institute in Peoria, Illinois. My enthusiasm for the position was the opportunity to contribute to an expansive two state health system bringing together 11 hospitals and the joy and adventure of living in the Midwest, a region of the country I had not experienced earlier. As the chief executive officer, I was responsible and accountable for overseeing strategic initiatives, marketing and branding, clinical and operational design, capital and operating budgets, development and delivery, and consolidation and integration of the Illinois Neurological Institute and neuroscience service line across the OSF HealthCare System. These experiences led me to further develop my leadership skills into the 9-Cs: how I can collaborate, cooperate, coordinate, consolidate, communicate, and convince our team to create world-class neuroscience services and define what we are focusing on improving clinical outcomes, research, and education. Additionally, while serving as a coach, having courage to make difficult decisions in these challenging healthcare times and encouraging everyone to contribute. I learned that coaching and instilling courage in others is essential to help others achieve their goals.

When I was the chief executive officer of the OSF HealthCare Illinois Neurological Institute, I was given the opportunity to learn about my strengths, weaknesses, and leadership potential through the two-year OSF ministry leadership formation program. From this two-year journey of personal reflection, I decided to tell my story to raise awareness of mental health and remove the stigma so that others would have the courage to seek help. I also had the opportunity to reflect on the other important experiences that had changed my life.

In June 2018, I was recruited by Michigan State University in East Lansing, Michigan, to help develop a safer and healthier campus. As a former high school and college football player and now an endurance ultra-runner, I am passionate about caring for young people, athletes, and their families, including creating support systems that emphasize performance, wellness, health, and safety.

All these titles and degrees do not mean much if I cannot make a difference in someone's life or give back to society. In the forthcoming pages, I will describe my relationships with Jake Anderson, Blake Nordstrom, Ryan Kupfer and his parents, Matthew Metcalf and his parents, and Ed Rapp, which have all shaped my life and given me the courage to tell my story.

FINDING MY WAY

Through endurance ultra-running, friendships, and other self-coping skills, I control my negativity, but it is an ongoing struggle (see Image #1). Like any disease, the first step is to diagnose the problem so we can do something about it. As a neurosurgeon, I have put other people's lives, limbs, and organs at risk for over 20 years. What keeps me up at night is not the hundreds of children that had a great outcome, but the couple of bad outcomes every year where I made an honest error or the disease won. I started my practice 20 years ago, and I have over 40 children that I blame myself for not helping. I constantly beat myself up, and all this increasing stress has taken a toll on my mental and physical well-being.

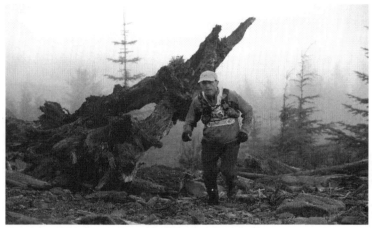

Image #1: Running the Capital Peak 50 mile race on April 26, 2014, in Capital Forest, Washington (Photo by Glenn Tachiyama).

When I was a neurosurgery resident at the trauma hospital, I used to say, "The best admission is a dead one." Looking back, these words were hurtful. I lost empathy and viewed patients as objects rather than human beings. Seeing someone die every day and the pain experienced by their loved ones was completely overwhelming. We all express our insecurities; it is how we deal with them and find inner peace that is key. Since my suicide attempt, I have found inner peace through endurance ultra-running races, which are running events longer than a marathon: 50 kilometer, 50 mile, 100 kilometer, and 100 mile races. I find that ultra-races are just like the "Hills of Life" (see Image #2). You need to prepare–start–work as a team–stay focused–finish. Training and competing in ultra-running races continues to help me learn self-coping skills to overcome mental and physical challenges. When running through the mountains on rugged terrain during an ultra-race, I find that mental toughness is more important than physical endurance.

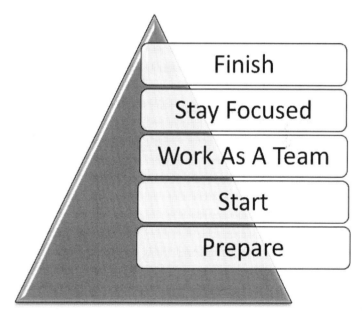

Image #2: Hills of Life.

Long distance ultra-running is what keeps me connected with helping others, both spiritually and emotionally. It has helped me cope with adversity and learn about myself in more ways than I dreamed possible. During some of the most difficult times of my life, I have found hope, healing, and purpose on the trails. I am at total peace on the trails (see Image #3). I still struggle with my demons, and my pain from depression is worse than a physical injury. When I cycle into a depressed state, I cannot sleep, think clearly, make decisions, or eat. I also have shoulder pain and have bad thoughts. I have realized that it is how one handles setbacks and failure that is key to developing resiliency and well-being.

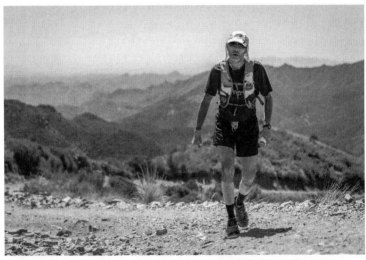

Image #3: Running the Crown King Scramble 50 kilometer race on March 30, 2019 in Crown King, Arizona (Photo by Jubilee Paige).

MENTAL HEALTH STATISTICS

The World Health Organization constitution states: "Health is a state of complete physical, mental and social well-being and not merely the absence of disease or infirmity."

An important implication of this definition is that mental health is more than just the absence of mental disorders or disabilities. Mental health is a state of well-being in which an individual realizes their own abilities, copes with the normal stresses of life, works productively, and makes a contribution to their community (1).

Suicide is the 10th leading cause of death in the United States and the second leading cause of death for those 10–34 years of age. Every 40 seconds, a person dies by suicide somewhere in the world. A quarter of people know of someone who died from suicide, and 40 percent know of someone that attempted. In the United States, there are 1.4 million suicide attempts annually. In 2017, 129 suicides were averaged per day, and 47,173 Americans died by suicide, 69.7 percent being white men (2). This should bring pause to anyone reading this. Suicide is a public health crisis, and we must remove the stigma so that those with mental health concerns seek help.

If you are experiencing suicidal thoughts, please call the National Suicide Prevention Lifeline at 1-800-273-8255.

Mental health can affect anyone. One in five struggles from mental illness—they may be an athlete, doctor, lawyer, cook, professor, sanitation worker, grocery worker, utility worker, musician, teacher, anyone. According to the World

Health Organization, depression is the leading cause of disability worldwide and greater than 300 million people of all ages suffer. In the United States, the breakdown of mental illness has been shown to be 18.1 percent anxiety, 6.9 percent depression, 2.6 percent bipolar disorder, and 1.1 percent schizophrenia (3). Serious mental illness costs America $193.2 billion in lost earnings per year (3). According to the Commonwealth Fund, the United States spends more on health care yet has the lowest life expectancy and the highest suicide rates (13.9 deaths/100,000 population) among 10 other high-income countries (4).

It has been said that one-third of college students experience depression, anxiety, or other mental health concerns; only 30 percent of those and 10 percent of athletes seek help. In my role as the interim director of athletic medicine at Michigan State University, I learned that mental health is the number priority for the National Collegiate Athletic Association and that suicide is the third leading cause of death, followed by accidents and cardiac failure. It has been suggested that 40 percent of NBA players have mental health concerns, yet less than 5 percent seek help. Thank you to Kevin Love and DeMar DeRozan, who have come forward to tell their story and raise awareness. According to the Healthy Minds Study (5), an annual web-based survey of 155,026 college students from 196 campuses, the percentage of students with a diagnosed mental health condition increased from 22 percent (2007) to 36 percent (2017), and the rate of treatment increased from 19 percent (2007) to 34 percent (2017).

From these preceding statistics and the implications of social distancing and isolation that the world is experiencing during the current COVID-19 pandemic in 2020, we must all agree that it is more important than ever to raise awareness of mental health and remove the stigma so that one has the courage to seek help to lead a more healthy, peaceful, and purposeful life.

STUTTERING

The most important aspect of my life that has kept me grounded and humble is managing my stuttering. Everyone has some problems, but it is how you deal with adversity and pick yourself up that matters most. Life is challenging, and everyone faces setbacks, but you need to keep moving forward. There is no doubt that being a stutterer has created anxiety and increased stress in my life.

My life as a stutterer involves constant fear and extreme frustration! The physical sensation feels like a tightening of my stomach and being unable to speak smoothly when I really want to! People must be laughing and thinking "what a dumb and stupid fool!" These are some of the feelings I encounter through my life as a stutterer. My problem is not unique. In fact, based on the evidence now available, it is widely agreed that the overall prevalence of stuttering is 0.7 percent among the general populations of all ages and occurs three to four times as often in males than in females (6).

I was born "handicapable" in verbally expressing myself, and as far back as I can remember, there was never a time when I did not stutter. Before learning to control my stuttering, my daily life was frustrating, miserable, and lonely at times. Just imagine not being able to talk to someone and when trying, sounding like a skipping record on a turntable. My stuttering generally involves the interruption of my speech flow by hesitations, unpredictable difficulties in progressing from one sound to the next with repetition, prolonging of sounds, avoiding difficult words, and debilitating blocking—trying to speak but cannot, because I have no air flow.

My resulting symptoms of stuttering when speaking to others include facial grimacing, looking away, closing my eyes, and contorting my body in an enormous effort to move from one word to the next. My stuttering problem is unique in that I rarely stutter when I am alone, singing, speaking in unison, or speaking in front of large groups. However, I have difficulty in talking one-on-one and, especially, talking on the telephone. It is very frustrating that I stutter in only some situations and not in others. Whenever I approach a speech situation and begin to speak, I must deal with the anxieties and uncertainties that affect my speech.

Memories of situational fears (e.g., when I'm introducing myself), trying to say difficult words or sounds (e.g., when I'm saying words beginning with "t," "n," "k," and "g"), and talking to an authoritative person (e.g., when I'm speaking with a girlfriend's father) increase my anxiety, anticipation, and apprehension about stuttering. In fact, I feel as conditioned as Pavlov's dog to go into a major block whenever I am in one of my "stuttering situations." I react to old memories of repeated speech failure in these arduous and fearful situations.

Interesting examples on what I did to not stutter included saying another word when I meant to say something different. For example, I might say "I went away for Christmas to G," filling in with the word "Gettysburg," when I really meant to say exotic "Guadeloupe." I also used to say sentences backward. For example, I used to say, "Mark, the small park we go, today?" instead of "Mark, do you want to go to the small park, today?"

Other stutterers and I manage our lives fairly well and have learned to cope with the fear, despair, humiliation, and frustration that accompany ourselves every time we stutter. According to the Stuttering Foundation of America (Memphis, TN), there are many talented and successful people who stutter, including: King George VI, Prime Minister Winston Churchill, physicist Albert Einstein, scientist Charles Darwin, actress Marilyn Monroe, legendary Chicago Bulls star Bob Love, former Vice President and now President Joseph Biden, actress Nicole Kidman, professional golfer Tiger Woods, actor Bruce Willis, TV host Mike Rowe, pop singer Marc Anthony, businessman Jack Welch, national news correspondent Byron Pitts, world-renowned TV correspondent John Stossel, Oscar and Grammy winner Carly Simon, NBA star Kenyon Martin, NBA Hall of Famer and NBC Sports commentator Bill Walton, country music artist Mel Tillis, major league baseball player Johnny Damon, and many more. People who react badly to stuttering are not usually deliberately unkind. They respond to their fear that they cannot cope with the unfamiliar situation and tend to copy the behavior of others toward people with noticeable disabilities. Stuttering is just not part of someone's usual encountering experiences; thus, society finds it hard to understand and accept stuttering.

WHAT THERAPY FINALLY BROUGHT MY STUTTER UNDER CONTROL?

After many unsuccessful attempts to control my stuttering with many compassionate and dedicated speech therapists, I was fortunate to work with a speech therapist in junior high school who acquainted me with the regulated breathing approach for stuttering introduced by Azrin and Nunn (7). The stated aim of this therapy was to develop a procedure that would abolish my stuttering in most of my everyday "stuttering situations." My program generally was divided into the following four progressive segments: (1) finding out when and why I stutter, (2) speech training, (3) training for generalization, and (4) home assignments.

(1) FINDING OUT WHEN AND WHY I STUTTER

First, I reviewed retrospectively, cognitively and verbally the development of my stuttering. In therapy, I recalled and verbalized the unpleasantness caused by my stuttering up to that time. This kind of initiation of therapy strengthened my motivation and determination to carry out future therapeutic measures. I was then asked to describe my stuttering reactions and my concomitant symptoms as precisely as possible. This included instances that triggered my stuttering, such as the words that caused special difficulties, the specific situations or contact with specific persons that were conducive to stuttering, and other stuttering situations I previously described.

Through this process, I came to know that my stuttering depended on a variety of conditions, for which I hoped to be better prepared for in the future. Based on the assumption that stuttering is generally bound up with a state of heightened tension, I was also instructed in techniques of relaxation. When speaking, I worked on achieving body relaxation as soon as possible, enabling me to breathe deeply, slowly, and regularly. The self-instruction of saying "I am completely calm and relaxed" whenever I spoke helped relieve my tension.

(2) SPEECH TRAINING

The chief objective of this next part of therapy was to establish a breathing pattern of behavior that would alleviate my urge to stutter when in a difficult "stuttering situation." If a symptom occurred, I was instructed to stop talking immediately, exhale deeply, and then inhale slowly. This consciously relaxed the upper part of my body and the muscles of my neck, while saying "I am completely calm and relaxed." Then, I consciously formulated a word to be spoken, exhaled a little bit of air out, and spoke by prolonging the first letter or syllable of the word very softly, freely, and slowly while maintaining eye contact and having confidence.

From the above set of rules, I basically learned how to breathe a certain way when speaking, which was extremely frustrating and sometimes very lonely, as one would imagine.

(3) TRAINING FOR GENERALIZATION

In the next step of my therapy, I constantly practiced my new speaking and breathing techniques. I consciously went into many of my difficult "stuttering situations" and performed my new breathing pattern and behavior to help alleviate my fear and regain confidence. In addition, I practiced my new breathing pattern by reading passages from children's books. At first, I paused after each word while being coached by my therapist to relax and take a deep breath. After achieving fluency at this level, the number of speech units spoken between breaths slowly increased (i.e., after every second word, every third word, and etc.). Moreover, on the certain sounds and words that I required a great amount of effort, I stopped and repeated them deliberately at various places in the sentences to gain confidence. It is important to note that my speech therapist was constantly helping and instilling confidence in me to speak without a stutter while concentrating on my new breathing pattern. Furthermore, the encouragement, strength, and support I received from my speech therapist, family, and friends were very similar to the encouragement, strength, and support that I show toward my patients and their families.

(4) HOME ASSIGNMENTS

After the above described training sessions, in which I went one hour per week for six months, I was given a few home assignments to maintain my fluency. These assignments included a 15-minute relaxation exercise every day, in which I practiced my breathing pattern on certain difficult words and on the pronunciation of the English vowels (i.e., a, e, i, o, u).

Additionally, a speech contract was drawn up between my therapist and I, which consisted of me promising to always use and practice my new breathing pattern and to relax and become more confident when speaking. In addition, in high school, college, and medical school, I always wrote the letters "PR" for "powerful rest" on my notebooks to remind myself to use my breathing pattern, as a constant reminder to speak passively, softly, and slowly (see Image #4).

In short, this speech program involved breathing, attitude, relaxation, and desensitization methods that helped bring my stutter mostly under control. I continue to maintain my fluency every day by practicing my learned techniques.

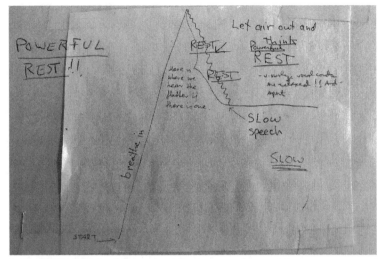

Image #4: This is the image I first created over 30 years ago, and I still use it today.

Stuttering is an enigma! No one knows what causes it and why different therapeutic approaches benefit some stutterers but not others. Although stuttering may sound gloomy, it is not, really, because most people who stutter like me can—if they cooperate fully—be taught to control it to the extent that it is no longer a social embarrassment for them.

I will always be grateful to my many speech therapists, family, and friends for their compassion, perceptiveness, and unswerving dedication in helping me learn to communicate without major interruptions to express my thoughts and feelings much more freely. I will also be forever grateful to them for still calling attention to my new breathing pattern whenever I forget to apply it when I talk, in addition to their constant support and encouragement in always reminding me to relax and breathe deeply and talk slowly when I do stutter. Although I do occasionally stutter, I have benefited greatly from the will power, courage, and determination I gained to succeed and learned not to quit. Controlling my stuttering helped me appreciate the need to motivate and help others overcome challenges. In fact, through the sensitivity and warmth of my dedicated speech therapists, I gained a fascination with how rehabilitation can make a person feel comfortable with themselves and with others around, which was one of my main inspirations on choosing a career in medicine.

In surviving childhood, adolescence, and adulthood with a speech impediment so far, I have seen some of the darkest and the brightest sides of humanity, and I must say the bright side reigns supreme indeed! Stuttering has truly taught me how we can learn from our failures by working hard and having a well-executed plan. It has kept me humble; when I become overconfident, my stuttering brings me down to reality.

Part II

Learn (from failures)

"There are no problems, only opportunities
for growth."

—Rebbetzin Dena Weinberg

I would not be where I am today if I did not fail and take the learnings of my failures to continuously improve my physical, mental, and relationship health. I always argue that being mentally healthy is just as important as being physically healthy. It is important to turn your failures and obstacles into opportunities for success. One's ability to continually self-improve, receive critical feedback, and develop resilience is essential to growing and achieving goals. Resilience is defined as the acquired ability to recover, adapt, and grow from stress. Developing a new mindset of coping and self-care skills to manage one's stress is essential to being resilient. Coping and self-care skills include time management; goal setting; positive self-talk; relaxation-mindfulness techniques; imagery-visualization techniques; and healthy sleep, eating, and exercise habits. For example, in the previous section, I describe my stuttering journey and how relaxation techniques helped bring my stutter mostly under control.

Showing kindness, compassion, love, and respect for yourself and others are critical to having healthy relationships. We must all be like bamboo—able to bend easily and snap back in shape without breaking—to build resilience. Social isolation is not the answer, and we need to have healthy relationships to avoid burnout. Others will perceive you as you see yourself; thus, it is important to see yourself positively with a "Be Your Best" attitude.

As I transitioned into different phases of my life from high school to college to medical school to residency to my current job, I learned to be cognizant of these transitions which can lead to stress and anxiety. Stress is defined as pushing past one's perceived limits. Stress, anxiety, depression, sleep difficulties, and debt are all impediments to success. In the age of social media, everyone has a perfect life, and there are expectations to perform, be perfect, and be tough. I thought climbing the ladder from high school to college to medical school was all-important, as each rung of the ladder would lead me closer to success and ultimate happiness. However, I had this fear that I needed to accomplish so many things prior to age 50, as I did not think I would live past 50. Once I turned 50, I realized that I was not happy, even though I achieved much academic and professional success. I realized I needed to have healthy relationships with my family so that I could recharge.

Besides my countless learnings from being a stutterer, as described previously, the following are the four most important lessons that I hope to instill in you so you can achieve academic success and life-long wellness:

1. Passion and purpose
2. Failure
3. Communication and teamwork
4. Relationships

PASSION AND PURPOSE

"I'd tell men and women in their
mid-twenties not to settle for a job or
profession or even a career. Seek a calling."

—Phil Knight

It has been shown that those who have purpose and passion are happier, do better, and have higher performance, leading to improved health and well-being. You cannot work hard and be passionate if you do not have personal peace and supportive relationships outside work. Purposeful and meaningful work adds value to your life. Viktor Frankel, a Holocaust survivor and well-known neurologist and psychiatrist, describes in his book *Man's Search for Meaning* that finding meaning in life is the most powerful motivation force in humans (1). Being appreciated and having input in decisions that affect your work (e.g., over work schedule) are also critical to your sense of worth.

You need to strive for academic excellence and accountability. You need to develop your growth mindset of being passionate about what you do in your work and personal life. Believe in your ideas, work to achieve your goals, and strive to reach your personal potential. People are different, and you need to live your life. Be positive toward yourself. You may not be perfect, but you know you are learning. Ask yourself: What is my passion? What makes me happy? What brings me joy? What makes me smile? What is important to me? What does success mean to me? What brings me peace? Is it exercising, gardening, praying, music, knitting, or reading? Are you mentally ready?

What are your motivators, challenges, strengths, and strategies to ensure success? Are your goals SMART (i.e., specific, measurable, attainable, relevant, and time-based)?

Education is knowledge, and knowledge is power.

How would you describe yourself when you are at your best? Are you calm, caring, compassionate, and courageous; balanced, impactful, and learning; or in-the-zone, productive, and reliable?

Mastery is hard work and painful at times; therefore, we often do not try new things for the fear of the unknown.

Effort is one of those things that gives meaning to your life. Effort means you care about something, something is important to you, and you are willing to work for it.

Commit yourself to be passionate and value things and then work toward that goal. Bring your best self to the things that matter most to you!

FAILURE

> "A righteous man falls down seven times
> and gets up."

> —King Solomon, Proverbs, 24:16.

Have a growth mindset. Embrace failure and learn from it so you make appropriate changes to optimize your performance. You cannot be afraid to fail. If you are not failing, you are not taking enough risk. Failure means you are growing, finding personal strength, gaining appreciation, forming deeper relationships, discovering more meaning in life, and seeing new possibilities. We all fail and make mistakes. It is how we rebound and continuously improve that is key to being resilient. Failing means you are like a caterpillar, transforming to a butterfly and getting stronger.

I would like to share with you a few of my significant failures that changed my life from my time at Cornell University and Columbia University College of Physicians & Surgeons. In my first semester at Cornell, I was taking a chemistry course that all premedical students take as it was a weed-out course (i.e., if you do not do well, you will have difficulty in other premedical courses). I was on track for a C grade, so I went to my lab preceptor for guidance a few weeks prior to the final exam. He said to me, "Do you really want to be a doctor?" These words affected me, and I studied and studied for two weeks and obtained an A on the final exam and a B+ in the class. This experience gave me the confidence I needed to continue to work hard to achieve my passion and dream of becoming a physician.

Another example was in my first semester at Columbia. I did okay but not great, as I was intimidated by many of my classmates who came from Harvard, Yale, and Princeton. I had not gained admission in these schools and felt inferior. However, after much soul searching, I learned that we are all humans, and if you have the passion and work hard, you can achieve anything you want.

Having the ability to find meaning in failures enables one to reflect and have a transformative experience to learn and improve. Remember, it is not how you start but how you learn along the journey to finish strong that matters.

As a neurosurgeon, I continually learn the most from children I have had the privilege to treat over the last 20 years. The children that keep me up at night are those whom I hurt through an honest mistake or could not help as they had a devastating disease with no available treatment. It is not like the medical TV shows where medicine is glorified. However, it is a great privilege to take care of a child and their family in need, even though there is a tremendous amount of stress in doing so. I have come to see human suffering and triumphs at both extremes.

One child I had the privilege to care for at Johns Hopkins University Hospital was Ryan Kupfer, who showed me the healing power of prayer (see Image #5). The power of prayer in healing and recovery has always amazed me and has been confirmed many times over again in my career!

I remember being called in one Sunday afternoon for a nine-year-old child who was sitting and belted in the back seat when another car hit the family station wagon on their way to church. The child's mother and brother remarkably escaped with minor injuries—proof from the beginning that God was in control of the family's journey! However, Ryan sustained a severe brain injury in which I had little hope for recovery but performed an emergent brain operation by removing half his skull bone to relieve his increased brain pressures. After the operation, his brain pressures gradually dropped.

From the beginning and on many occasions thereafter, I observed his family, friends, and relatives in prayer. There was a deep and undeniable faith among them. Over the ensuing months, Ryan's parents and I had numerous interactions, as Ryan needed subsequent neurosurgery procedures. Prior to one of these procedures, Ryan's mom, Debbie, asked me, "Dr. Avellino, do you pray before you perform surgery?" I responded by pulling out the crucifix that I have worn around my neck for many years and, in showing her my cross, Ryan's mom was comforted. Over the ensuing months and years, Ryan has made a remarkable recovery, one that has surpassed most medical and human expectations. I thank God for giving us the wisdom and determination to persevere in these most "challenging" times of life, as we allow Him to guide us—both parents and surgeons—as instruments in His healing (2)! Further, Ryan was recently married in October 2020.

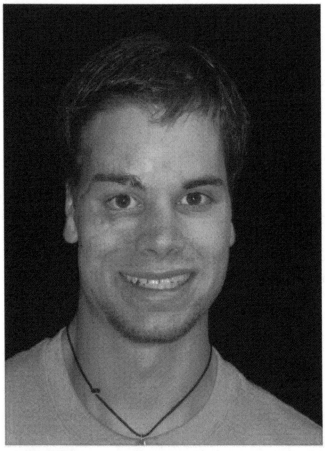

Image #5: Ryan is pictured here at age 25, 16 years after his initial injury (Photo by Debbie Kupfer).

Another child I had the privilege to care for was Matthew Metcalf. Matthew was a child who had acute lymphocytic leukemia when he was three years of age. He had chemotherapy and radiotherapy and was presumed cured until he relapsed at age 11, when I initially met him in 2003. His dad, Dan, was a long-haul truck driver and his mom, Sue, was an operating room nurse. Matthew had a brain tumor called a gliosarcoma, one of the most malignant types, and I could only remove 75 percent of it safely.

Unfortunately, the brain tumor recurred after four weeks. After talking with Matthew and his parents, I recommended another brain tumor operation. His parents stated that they are a spiritual family and knew another operation would not prolong his survival and declined. Instead, Matthew's dad decided to take Matthew on the road with him in order to visit many of his friends. As a young neurosurgeon, I struggled with their decision but respected their wishes. However, seven months later I heard that he passed, and I thought it was a peaceful way to die. After Matthew passed, I often thought of him and his parents and the lessons they taught me of spirituality and one's right to choose when to be with God. Dan, his dad, reminded me of my dad, who was an electrician, as both had blue-collar values.

In 2012, nine years after I first met Matthew, I had a life changing event: I received a copy of Dan's book, *He Chose Joy!: The Story of Matthew Metcalf*, and a heartfelt note that read " . . . our hope to help families know hope beyond illness . . . thank you" (3). I read Dan's book, was overcome with emotion, cried, and immediately reconnected with Matthew's family. At this time, I was struggling with depression and suicide and beginning to heal through ultra-running. Reconnecting with Dan and Sue has changed my life. They often crew for my ultra-races and have traveled to Vermont, Illinois, and Oregon to help me (see Image #6). In fact, the first 50 mile ultra-race I ran in Oregon, the Autumn Leaves 50/50, was the first race they crewed for me, and we raised over $8,000 to support the Matthew Metcalf Memorial Scholarship Fund at Life Christian Academy in Tacoma, Washington, to help a student in need to cover their tuition.

Connecting my self-coping skills of ultra-running with the purpose of helping another student in need where Matthew attended school helped me complete my first ultra-race. It is amazing that, nine years prior to receiving their book, I could not save their son, and now they have changed my life in more ways than they will ever know and helped me heal through my mental health struggles. I have told Matthew and his family's personal and touching story numerous times and always recommend Dan's book to others in time of need. Dan's book gives others hope in thanking God for giving us the wisdom and determination to persevere in our most challenging times of life. We allow Him to guide us to find hope even in the darkest moments for the lessons learned can give us insights on how to bring light to others.

Caring for Ryan and Matthew has reinforced my decision to be a physician, as helping others and their families through tragedies can both inspire and heal.

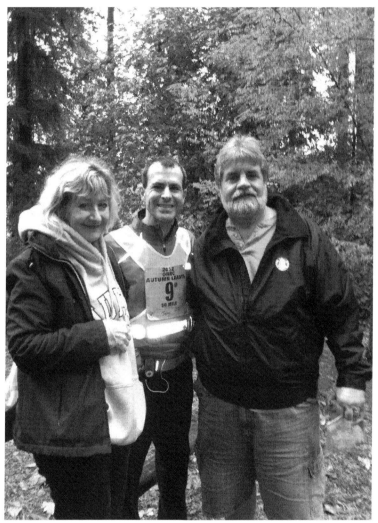

Image #6: Dan and Sue Metcalf crewing for my first ultra-race on October 27, 2012, the Autumn Leaves 50 mile in Champoeg State Park, St. Paul, Oregon (Photo by author).

COMMUNICATION AND TEAMWORK

"I will study and get ready, and someday
my chance will come ..."

—President Abe Lincoln

Many disagreements are caused by miscommunication. Think back on your disappointments? War, divorce, breakup with friends, decreased work satisfaction, losing a game, or not achieving your potential can all be attributed to not effectively communicating.

Being part of a team that achieves its goals is truly bigger than yourself. I played football in high school and college, and that taught me about teamwork and the thrill of succeeding. One of my biggest life joys was when, during my freshman year at Cornell, we won the Eastern Varsity Lightweight Football League World Championship. This experience changed my life; I learned that you will achieve more being a member of a team than performing alone in work and life.

As a neurosurgeon, I was fortunate to learn from the commercial fishing industry on how to translate that "my life is at risk" mentality to prevent mistakes from happening in healthcare. In 2009, I had the great privilege of working on the F/V *Miss Colleen*, a commercial salmon fishing gillnet boat in Bristol Bay, Alaska, with Nick Mavar, one of the deckhands of the Northwestern crab boat profiled on the Discovery show *Deadliest Catch*. In October 2019 and January 2021, I was also fortunate to be a deckhand on the F/V *Saga*, a commercial crab fishing boat in the Bering Sea with Captain Jake Anderson, who is also profiled on *Deadliest Catch*.

Cost, quality, and patient safety have been important issues facing US healthcare over the past decade, especially with the rollout of Obamacare and the present changes with Trumpcare. In 1999, the Institute of Medicine reported in its *To Err Is Human* publication that as many as 98,000 people die in any given year from preventable medical errors (4). In both the healthcare and commercial fishing industries, there is no room for error; giving the wrong medication or going overboard in rough seas can both lead to death. What then can the healthcare industry learn from the commercial fishing industry that would make healthcare safer and decrease healthcare costs? I believe effective communication and teamwork are the answers!

Fear . . . Anxiety . . . Discomfort . . . Am I going to die? Am I safe? Am I on the safest team? Do I trust my fellow team members? All these emotions come into play when one is facing their mortality when doing something dangerous.

Commercial fishing is known to be one of the most dangerous occupations in the world because of its high mortality rate. According to recent CDC and US Bureau of Labor Statistics reports, commercial fishing workers have the most dangerous job in the United States with 100 deaths per 100,000 workers—29 times higher than the average US workers (3.5 deaths/100,000 workers). *Deadliest Catch* has raised awareness of the Bering Sea crab fishing industry. There are similar stressors and risks with being a commercial fishing worker and being a surgeon. These crab fishing workers must meet their crab quota in a safe, timely manner while working in challenging weather on slippery decks with thousand-pound swinging crab pots, fearing the loss of their anticipated yearly income. Similarly, a healthcare worker must make quick decisions while working in a stressful environment.

Though seemingly dissimilar, whether a person is dealing with Mother Nature while navigating the frigid Bering Sea or with human nature inside the confines of a modern healthcare facility, commercial fishing and healthcare workers both have to be extremely cognizant of their surroundings as the slightest error or lapse in judgment may lead to devastating consequences and death. Although both industries require attention to detail, challenging work conditions, and long hours, the most important difference between healthcare and commercial fishing workers is that healthcare workers put other people's lives, limbs, and organs at risk, while commercial fishing workers put theirs at risk.

Without question, my work as a commercial fishing worker was physically and mentally agonizing—like running five ultra-races in a row—but I learned that safety is freedom! I also learned that to have effective teamwork, you need to develop compassionate and supportive relationships with your team; everyone must have each other's back to keep each other safe, as one mistake could lead to the death of the entire crew. Each team member knows one another's strengths and weaknesses to ensure safety and focus on completing the task at hand. Working on these fishing vessels, I was reminded that all the crew was at risk. Even though there were no work-hour restrictions, and we were fatigued, we were all extremely attentive of our surroundings, working as a high-level team. We each had specific roles and were in constant communication, so that we kept each other safe, leading to catching more crab and, in turn, reaping larger financial rewards. Importantly, all potential safety concerns on deck were immediately called out and corrected right away without any crew member feeling ashamed (e.g., when the hatch to the crab tank was not secured, crew members would yell "open hole on deck" to warn all other crew members of a potential hazard). There was no ego—the captain and crew were all on the same TEAM (i.e., together everyone achieves more). Similarly, in healthcare, all team members must communicate with each other to ensure we are doing the right operation or treatment while giving the correct medications on the right patient (5).

Over the past 10 years, Captain Jake Anderson and I have asked each other what makes a great captain, physician, and/or leader. We have agreed that the most successful leader wants all to succeed; is humble, respectful, and trustworthy; and leads by example. When fishing on the dangerous and unrelenting Bering Sea, one understands their mortality and that life is precious, fostering teamwork as they are constantly faced with death. Developing loving relationships, showing up, and knowing each team member's strengths and weaknesses is critical to combat loneliness and fear to keep everyone safe while focusing on the goal of catching your crab quota.

Captain Jake Anderson continues to be a close confidant of mine. Who would think that a brain surgeon and a commercial fisherman would have such a bond? Jake has been featured on *Deadliest Catch* since 2007. He is a fourth-generation fisherman. At 17 years of age, he was fishing salmon off Bristol Bay in Alaska; at 20, he was on a trawler processor; and at 25, he began pot fishing. Just one year later, he became a greenhorn on the F/V *Northwestern*, where he worked for the next six years. His hard work and charisma carried him from greenhorn to full-share deckhand to relief deck boss, under Captain Sig Hansen. In 2015, he took over as captain of the F/V *Saga*, and he immediately set about rebuilding the boat from the ground up, while fishing one of the largest king crab quotas in the fleet. He installed a new refrigeration system, cleaned fuel and water tanks, rebuilt all the boat's engines, repainted the boat with a new color scheme, fully upgraded the wheelhouse to improve efficiency and safety, and reconstructed the crane and most of the hydraulic system. However, the hardest thing to fix was the boat's reputation. Although Jake has experienced his fair-share of trials, he's also worked to overcome them. Since his sister's sudden death and his father's murder, Jake has matured—and aged—dramatically. He beat addiction in 2010, and his leadership continues to blossom, as he transforms the F/V *Saga* into a crab-catching machine that cements his place amongst the greats. In October 2019 and January 2021, I was fortunate to be a deckhand on the F/V *Saga*; I was in awe to see the person that Jake has become (see Images #7 and #8).

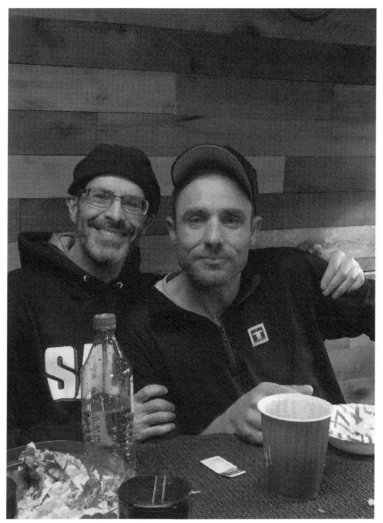

Image #7: Jake and I in the galley on the F/V *Saga* in October 2019 (Photo by author).

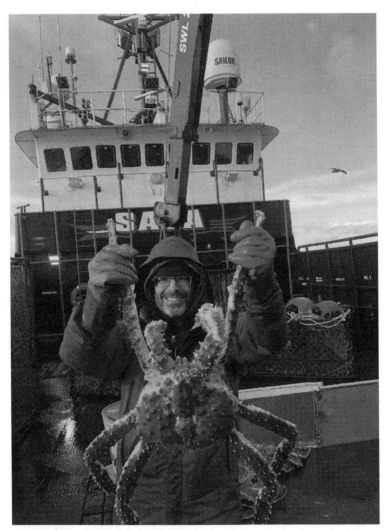

Image #8: I am holding a King Crab on the deck of the F/V *Saga* in October 2019 (Photo by author).

RELATIONSHIPS

"A setback is a setup for a comeback!"

—Ice Cube

Developing healthy relationships and having mentors to show you the way and bounce ideas off is essential to continually improving oneself. I often say that having supportive family, friends, and colleagues are more important than our accomplishments. Make as many friends as possible, as your success depends on it. Let me tell you about a few of my mentors: Dr. Andrew Frantz, Blake Nordstrom, and Ed Rapp. My first mentor was Dr. Andrew Frantz, the dean of admissions at Columbia University College of Physicians & Surgeons. I can honestly say that his belief in me was essential for me to not be intimidated by others and play my own game. He gave me the opportunity to attend Columbia when he accepted me on the spot two waitlists and three interviews later. My persistence and sending him a copy of my first book *So You Want To Be A Doctor?* enabled him to feel my passion of wanting to be a physician and the opportunity to attend Columbia (6). After he received a copy of my book, he invited me for a third interview, and after an hour of meeting him, he turned to me and asked, "Do you want to come here? Is it your first choice?"

I responded with an emphatic "yes" and said, "I was raised a few blocks from Columbia when I was a child and remember coming to the Columbia University Presbyterian Hospital emergency room, and I want to attend Columbia with all my passion."

He said, "You're accepted," and went into the next office to ask his assistant to type me an acceptance letter. I was moved to tears, and we hugged. We subsequently met every month while I attended Columbia, and his mentorship and friendship were invaluable to me. Another lesson I learned from Dr. Frantz was during my first year: I showed up to one of our monthly meetings unshaven and in sweatpants. He looked at me and said, "Tony, you are a doctor. You need to look and act like one, from now on. Go home, shave, dress, and come back." I did all that he asked and came back. This was a lesson I will never forget, as being a physician is an incredible privilege, and one must look the part, or your patient and their family will not take you seriously.

Another mentor during my University of Washington days was Blake Nordstrom, President of Nordstrom department stores. I reached out to Blake when I was a young attending at Seattle Children's Hospital and asked him to come to our clinics as I wanted to provide "Nordstrom-like healthcare." He wrote back and said, "I'm not qualified, as I'm only a shoe salesman, but I'm happy to meet." I invited Blake into our clinics to learn how to improve our patient and family experience. When a patient and their family come to see me, they're unhappy and sad, and I wanted them happy and satisfied when they left. I wanted them to have all their care coordinated: all their appointments, imaging, and lab work scheduled prior to leaving the clinic. I learned that at Nordstrom, the customer being most important and treating your employees well are keys to success. I learned that the Nordstrom cashier is the first and last person the customer sees, and they always need to smile and be nice, similar to our patient coordinators in healthcare. Further, he invited me multiple times to his department store reward events where I learned that being recognized among and in front of your peers is more important than monetary reward. Blake recently died in 2019 from cancer, and his smile, wisdom, and engaging personality will be missed by myself and many others.

Another mentor of mine was Ed Rapp, past group president for Caterpillar Inc. I met Ed in 2016, when he had recently returned to Peoria, Illinois, from working in Singapore for future leadership advancement. However, six months prior to his advancement, he was diagnosed with amyotrophic lateral sclerosis (ALS), also known as Lou Gehrig's disease, a specific disease that causes the death of neurons controlling voluntary muscles. Subsequently, he retired early and supported our research efforts when I worked at OSF HealthCare with significant philanthropy. He taught me more about achieving a more effective work-life balance then he will ever know, and I will share his three tools in the next section. I can honestly say that Ed is at total peace, living his life with God and still fighting to live a meaningful and purposeful life.

Part III

Heal (to achieve a healthier and more purposeful life)

"If you don't know what you're living for,
you haven't yet lived."

—Rabbi Noah Weinberg

My goal is to empower you with wellness tactics as you begin your healing journey into achieving optimum performance and a better work-life balance to lead a more healthy, peaceful, and purposeful life. It is important to have mental health, physical health, and relationship health so that one has a plan, enhanced energy, and stress tolerance. Having a plan is most essential for you to develop confidence to achieve your goals.

THE BRAIN AND STRESS RESPONSES

"To me, there are three things we all should
do every day. We should do this every day of
our lives. Number one is laugh. You should
laugh every day. Number two is think.
You should spend some time in thought.
And number three is, you should have your
emotions moved to tears, could be happiness
or joy. But think about it. If you laugh, you
think, and you cry, that's a full day. That's a
heck of a day. You do that seven days a week,
you're going to have something special."

—JIM VALVANO

I became a neurosurgeon, because I was fascinated with the brain, as we know very little about how the brain functions, especially about cognition and mental health. The nervous system contains the brain, spinal cord, and billions of nerve cells; it allows the human body to adjust to its outside environment. Your brain weighs only 3 pounds, continues to grow until 6 years of age, and makes up 2 percent of your human body weight. It has a texture like a very soft mushroom and Jell-O. Your brain is like a control room: it directs all your thinking, feeling, talking, and moving. It controls your body and mind!

The brain is enclosed within the skull and consists of the cerebrum, cerebellum, and brainstem. The cerebrum is the largest part and is composed of the right and left hemispheres.

Each hemisphere comprises the frontal, parietal, occipital, and temporal lobes. The frontal lobe controls personality, emotions, thinking, speech, and movement of one's limbs. The parietal lobe integrates sensory information and enables us to sense touch, pain, and temperature. The occipital lobe is important for vision. The temporal lobe works to understand language, memories, and hearing. The right side of the brain controls the left side of the body, and the left side of the brain controls the right side of the body. The cerebellum is located under the cerebrum and controls our balance and coordination. The brainstem connects the cerebrum and cerebellum with the spinal cord and controls our breathing, heart rate, digestion, and sleep/wake cycles (see Image #9).

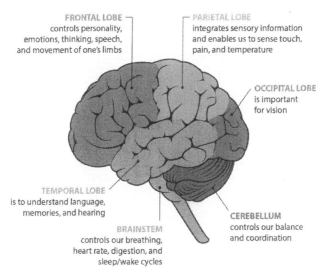

Image #9: The regions of the brain.

The amygdala, prefrontal cortex, and the hypothalamic–pituitary–adrenal axis are the parts of the brain that are responsible for our internal and external stress responses through activation of our hormonal and autonomic nervous systems. Stress is what we feel when we experience a threatening physical or emotional situation, which is manifest as increased heart rate, breathing, and anxiety. The amygdala is in the temporal lobe and detects physical and emotional stressors that activate the hypothalamic–pituitary–adrenal (HPA) axis. Once the HPA axis is activated, the hypothalamus sends a message to the pituitary gland which releases a hormone to the adrenal glands that release cortisol—the steroid hormone that influences our body responses to stress. The amygdala also shares connections to the prefrontal cortex which helps regulate the amygdala by controlling our stress responses (1). When I trained in neurosurgery at the University of Washington, I was fortunate to learn under Dr. George Ojemann, one of the pioneers in the study of human brain function during awake brain tumor and epilepsy operations. Presently, functional magnetic resonance imaging (fMRI) can map out motor, sensory, and language functions in humans by detecting changes in blood flow non-invasively (i.e., without opening the skull and placing electrodes on the brain). For example, fMRI has been used to study mindfulness and emotion regulation (2).

PERFORMANCE = SKILL – INTERFERENCE

> "Being a professional is doing the things
> you love to do, on the days you don't feel
> like doing them . . . "

—Julius Erving

I will argue that performance equals skill minus interference (3). If you are an athlete, scholar, musician, physician, teacher, janitor, painter, utility worker, or grocery worker, you can have all the skill in the world, but if you cannot manage your interference—if you are not mentally well, mentally prepared, doing purposeful work, happy and satisfied, in healthy relationships, and showing compassion toward yourself—you are not performing at your highest level. I know that my biggest mistakes in the operating room and in life were the ones when I had all the skill in the world, but my interferences prevented me from performing at the highest level. For example, I was thinking about an upcoming meeting, or my pager was going off, and I was not completely focused on the task at hand in the operating room. I say that being mentally ready, staying in the moment, feeling the now, and being passionate about what you are doing are essential to optimizing your performance.

In 1995, a research study was published on "mental readiness in surgeons and its links to performance excellence in surgery." It assessed mental, technical, and physical factors related to surgical excellence among surgeons performing high-mortality risk surgery (e.g., neurosurgery, cardiac surgery, and vascular surgery). In both athletes and surgeons, mental readiness was judged to be as important as technical readiness (4). I argue that mental readiness is more important than physical readiness. For example, in the NFL Super Bowl LI in 2017, didn't we all think that the New England Patriots would lose to the Atlanta Falcons? I argue that in the fourth quarter, Tom Brady, the quarterback of the New England Patriots, was mentally laser focused and brought his team back to win 34–28 in overtime after trailing by as many as 25 points during the third quarter. That is blocking out interference and performing at your highest level!

In *The Talent Code* (5), author Daniel Coyle outlines three parts to talent. He notes that in order to have optimum performance, you need deep practice, ignition, and master coaching. Deep practice requires commitment; you need to do something more than 10,000 hours (6). Ignition is motivational fuel. It is your passion that gives you the energy to be who you want to be. Master coaching helps you tap into your true desires and needs—it tailors to each student, telling them the right way to do something, the incorrect way, and the right way again. Combine deep practice, ignition, and master coaching—even for six minutes— and things begin to change to achieve talent. Who I am today, I attribute to my mentors and coaches I have had along my journey.

BURNOUT VERSUS WELL-BEING

"If you are not a better person tomorrow than you are today, what need have you for a tomorrow?"

—Rebbe Nachman

In 1982, Maslach described the Maslach Burnout Inventory Scale that assesses an individual's experience of burnout in the three dimensions of emotional exhaustion, depersonalization, and personal accomplishment. Emotional exhaustion refers to feeling tired and fatigued at work and being unable to recover from stress during your time off. Depersonalization is turning negative and cynical, developing callous and uncaring feelings (i.e., compassion fatigue), having trouble connecting with patients, and constantly blaming others. Reduced sense of personal accomplishment is lost confidence in your skills, and you start to believe that your work will not do any good (7).

We all need purposeful work, and when we are out of balance—meaning that our interference is greater than our skill—we do not optimize our performance, and we burn out. As a neurosurgeon, I say that our neuroscience work revolves around the brain health of our patients; part of maintaining their brain health is taking care of themselves and ourselves and striking a work-life balance. Treating ourselves kindly and compassionately, as we would treat a patient, can be vital to our general well-being and sense of happiness. There is science that demonstrates that love and affection saves lives. For example, babies cuddled in orphanages improve their survival and developmental quotient (8). In addition, in a rabbit atherosclerosis study, the rabbits were fed 2 percent cholesterol diets and were individually petted, held, talked to, and played with on a regular basis, and they had 60 percent less plaque buildup than those that were not (9).

Do you have effective work-life balance? Do you work seven days a week? If so, why? From the book of Genesis in the Bible, it says that "from a state of absolute nothingness, God created time, space, and the entire physical world—the process of creation took 6 days, and on the seventh day God rested." In *Gateway to Judaism* (10), author Rabbi Mordechai Becher notes that the Shabbat is the day of rest with spiritual and physical peace. He also notes that stopping each day to appreciate every aspect of our existence enables us to achieve greater happiness and be more content in life. Do you take a pause to recharge? Having the skills to recharge and relieve stress is essential to optimize your performance.

In *Healing Physician Burnout* (11), authors Quint Studer and George Ford describe the following factors that contribute to physician burnout: accelerating changes in the healthcare environment, practical hurdles, psychological challenges, organizational structure changes, and training challenges. These factors can also apply to other professions besides healthcare. Healthcare environmental factors include the escalating healthcare spending of 17.7 percent GDP or $11,172 per person in 2018 (12), value-based purchasing and new delivery models, and changing patient expectations. With the extraordinary amount of money we are spending, I ask, are we providing the very best health-care in the United States? I and others argue that there is too much waste within our healthcare system. Practical hurdles include mounting bureaucracy and regulations. Physicians feel overworked and sleep deprived, and there is little time with patients and too much doing everything else (e.g., using a user-unfriendly electronic medical record). Psychological challenges physicians face include missed important per-sonal events, loss of control, rapid pace of change, heavy debt, and stress related to uncertainty around the prognosis that we give our patients. Organizational structure changes have led to lack of leadership and the requirement of team-work skills not learned in medical school. Training challenges include the increasing use of the internet for information and changing attitudes on work-life balance. Without a healthy work-life balance, we are at risk of burnout. Burnout can lead to impaired judgment, lack of attention to detail, and com-munication failure, all of which impact the quality and safety of patient care. Symptoms include anxiety, depression and suicidal ideation, insomnia, apathy and loneliness, marital and family stress, anger and boundary issues, overeating, and addiction and substance abuse—any of which can lead to dissatisfaction with work-life balance and, ultimately, pro-fessionals leaving their careers.

Physicians are twice as likely to be dissatisfied with their work-life balance than the average working adult. Medical students' rate of depression is 15–30 percent higher than that of the general public. In 2017, 39.8 percent of physicians reported that they were burned out, compared to 28.1 percent of other US workers (13). We have over one million physicians in the United States and therefore over 400,000 are burned out. This is a true public health crisis. Physicians are more than twice as likely to commit suicide than the general population. Each year, roughly 300–400 physicians commit suicide. In a 2015 Mayo Study (14), 7 percent of employed physicians between ages of 29–65 considered suicide in the past 12 months (compared to 4 percent of other workers). Female physicians are 2.5–4 times as likely as women in other occupations to commit suicide. According to a 2011 Cejka study (15), the burnout turnover costs were $1,262,297 per physician (i.e., lost downstream revenue of $990,034, recruitment expenses of $61,200, and investment in bringing up to speed of $211,063). In 2019, a cost-consequence analysis model study showed that approximately $4.6 billion in costs related to physician turnover and reduced clinical hours is attributable to burnout each year in the United States (16).

WORK-LIFE BALANCE

"Life is like riding a bicycle: to keep your
balance you must keep moving."

—Albert Einstein

As you journey through the different stages of life, your interests, passion, purpose, and goals evolve, and you must adapt, recover, and move forward in a healthy way. Depending on the year you were born, your cultural beliefs may be different than other generations (i.e., Boomers 1946–1964, Generation X 1965–1976, Generation Y or Millennials 1977–1995, Generation Z or Centennials 1994–2010). Having holistic physical and mental health in today's fast paced world is essential.

As I speak with many students and colleagues about achieving effective work-life balance, I always ask three questions: Do you drive your kids to school once a week? Do you see your grandkids once a week? Do you do something that brings you joy once a week? These are powerful questions that bring emotional responses as, at the end of our life, most would agree that family is most important.

The following are three tools I learned from Ed Rapp that I would like to share with you to achieve better work-life balance and lead a healthy, peaceful, and purposeful life:

1. Make a plan
2. Improve efficiency
3. Be a corporate athlete

(1) MAKE A PLAN

Having a plan is most essential for your overall success and well-being. It starts with what is your personal why or life vision. Is it based on self-esteem, honesty, faith, ethics, competitive spirit, respect, and/or responsibility? What inspires you to action? I never had a personal "why" or life vision until I was 50 years of age and met Ed Rapp. My personal why or life vision is "to be the best friend, dad, and spouse to make this world a better place." What is yours?

Each week, you should look at and set your calendar with all the things you want to do in the upcoming week. For example, scheduling time for family, hobbies, exercise, and others are important; if they are not in your calendar, these times are not protected and will be filled up with other, less important things. Having the ability to say "no" without explanation is important, as you need to prioritize your schedule so that you have time to recharge and promote recovery. Saying yes to all actually means saying no to other things that may be more important. Most importantly, having them scheduled in your calendar enables others to know you are not available at these times. I was an awful father—something I am not proud of—until I met Ed Rapp. I learned that scheduling within my calendar to drive my kids to school once a week as well as having breakfast or working out with my son for an hour every Sunday, having dinner with my daughter once a week for an hour, and having coffee with my wife for 30 minutes every two weeks was essential for me to recharge and stay connected with those I treasure, enabling me to be happier and more productive.

When I was the chief executive officer of the OSF Illinois Neurological Institute, I learned after a year that I was burning out my co-workers with my expectations that were not conducive to having a productive and engaged team. Thus, we created the "Avellino Team: Work-Life Parameters," which were:

- No expectation of an immediate response to emails evenings, weekends or vacation
- No more than one early morning meeting (before 7:00 a.m.) per week
- No more than one late night meeting (after 5:00 p.m.) per week
- No early and late meetings on same day
- No more than two mandatory after-hours activities per month
- Recruitment dinners are a priority
- Events are optional

These work-life parameters were important to our team. For example, if you are a mother or father who needs to drive and pick up your kids from school and activities, it is important to have a defined schedule, and it would be challenging for you to attend an early and late meeting on the same day. Further, after we rolled out and communicated our work-life parameters, we found that our team worked more efficiently—not harder—and had more joy and effective work-life balance. In fact, we increased our US News & World Report rankings for neurology and neurosurgery programs from #316 in 2015 to #84 in 2016 to #56 in 2017, and our net revenue, contribution margin, and total hospital encounters all increased significantly. Having a happy, healthy, and engaged staff are important to achieve one's organization goals.

The "Life Balance Sheet" is a tool I use with others to develop their one-, three-, and five-year personal and financial goals to allow them to continually learn, improve, and grow (see Image #10). At this time, I encourage you to write down your personal and financial goals using this tool within the diagram.

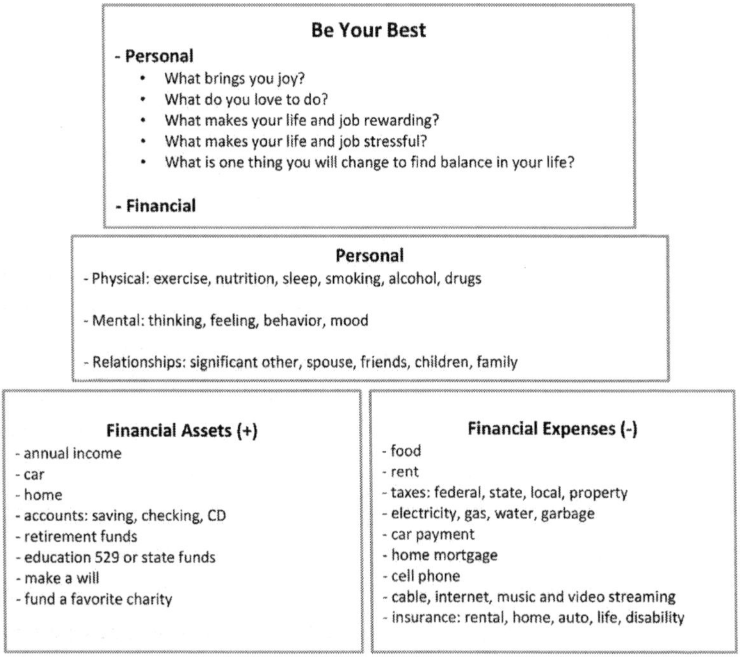

Be Your Best

- **Personal**
  - What brings you joy?
  - What do you love to do?
  - What makes your life and job rewarding?
  - What makes your life and job stressful?
  - What is one thing you will change to find balance in your life?

- **Financial**

Personal

- Physical: exercise, nutrition, sleep, smoking, alcohol, drugs

- Mental: thinking, feeling, behavior, mood

- Relationships: significant other, spouse, friends, children, family

Financial Assets (+)
- annual income
- car
- home
- accounts: saving, checking, CD
- retirement funds
- education 529 or state funds
- make a will
- fund a favorite charity

Financial Expenses (-)
- food
- rent
- taxes: federal, state, local, property
- electricity, gas, water, garbage
- car payment
- home mortgage
- cell phone
- cable, internet, music and video streaming
- insurance: rental, home, auto, life, disability

Image #10: Life Balance Sheet.

(2) IMPROVE EFFICIENCY

The goal is not working harder but smarter and more efficiently so you have more purposeful, productive, joyful and meaningful work. It is important to give yourself time to slow down, pause, rest, and be present. Further, having the ability to pause every month for 15 minutes to assess where you are physically and mentally in your work and personal life will bring you better focus and clarity.

Some efficiencies to consider are:

a. *Exercising*, feeding your pet, and engaging your family prior to starting your workday.

b. *Email* is good and bad: good as it enables all to have rapid access to messaging, but bad as it creates more work. I let my team know that short responses are key. If the email is more than a few sentences, I am not going to read it; it is better to call me. Further, how many times are you "cc'ed" on emails and, at end of day, you have many emails with everyone cc'ing each other emails with little substance? Thus, if you need to respond, only respond to those that need to know. Also, checking email two or three times a day enables you to focus on other things without constant distractions. Remember, performance equals skill minus interference!

c. *Technology* is changing so rapidly these days that using it effectively to your advantage is key. For example, smartphones from Apple and Android have many apps that can interrelate and make your life easier and more efficient. Using your smartphones in a healthy way is key. For example, when you go on vacation, do you take your smartphone and answer work emails? Why? It is important to disconnect and recharge so you are refreshed when you return to work. Further, there are apps to help you shop, prepare meals, and walk your pet, making your life more efficient and balanced. Seek these out and use them!

d. *Meetings* are critical to have if you need to make a decision or develop action plans. However, how many meetings have you gone to that go on for over 90 minutes, there is lots of spin, and nothing is accomplished? Having meetings for only 30 minutes is key, provided all are prepared. For example, if someone wants a meeting, I ask for the information to be sent three days prior regarding the decision points and action plans that are to be achieved. If all are prepared, the work is completed, and one can move forward to other strategic initiatives. Most importantly, meetings need to start and end on time. If you are a mother or father who need to pick up your children, it is important to not be delayed, and meetings that run late create an enormous amount of anxiety and anger. I know that after an hour, I'm not listening anymore.

e. *Simplify* your life. Bundle tasks if you can. For example, if you have the means to offload or outsource some chores like cleaning, lawncare, or weekly meal preparation, then it may be cheaper and more efficient to have someone else do them. However, if cleaning brings you joy and peace, then do it. No size fits all, and you must write down, put in your calendar, discuss, and communicate your plans to all!

(3) BE A CORPORATE ATHLETE

"The Making of a Corporate Athlete" by Jim Loehr and Tony Schwartz in the January 2001 *Harvard Business Review* uses the term "corporate athletes," in which they describe the "performance pyramid." They describe that high performance is achieved by having one's physical, emotional, mental, and spiritual capacities optimized (17).

Having a healthy mind, a healthy body, and healthy relationships is critical for one to recharge and to recover. Having enjoyment, happiness, and fun in your life is key to developing coping mechanisms to continually improve. Acknowledging the need to self-improve to minimize your interferences and maximize your performance is key. Managing stress and relieving anxiety to decrease your interferences must be a habit with no excuses—you must love to do it.

The most important lesson I learned from Ed Rapp is that "you get to choose what type of day you will have." If you wake up in the morning upset with your significant other, spouse, friend, mother, father, pet, children, or others, you will take this anger to work, which will lead you to be unpleasant with your fellow workers and your day will be ruined. This negativity drains your energy and increases your heart rate, blood pressure, and stress levels—all leading to your frustration, anger, and suboptimal performance. You have a choice to release your negativity. Thus, please promise me that, going forward, you say each morning, "Today will be a great day!" You need to smile and spread positivity!

Some stress management techniques that you can explore to achieve better focus, confidence, energy, and recovery are:

a. *Sleep*: I argue that sleep is the most important thing you can do to increase your performance, stamina, and recovery. Obtaining 7–9 hours of sleep each night with a consistent wake-up and bedtime is important to optimize your body to recover and heal (18).

b. *Exercise:* Having a healthy body is key to having a healthy brain. According to the current Department of Health and Human Services recommendations, most healthy adults should do 150–300 minutes a week of moderate aerobic activity or 75–150 minutes a week of vigorous aerobic activity or an equivalent combination of moderate and vigorous aerobic activity per week (19). Taking 15-minute walks twice a day to feel the now and be present can be therapeutic.

c. *Nutrition:* Having a healthy diet and staying hydrated are critical to perform at your highest level. For example, when I was starting out in endurance ultra-running, I sustained stress fractures, as I realized that my diet was not optimum; I was consuming too much sugar and not enough protein for my body to recover. I realized that eating more protein and less carbohydrates was key to satisfying my hunger throughout the day and maximizing my recovery. Eating a well-balanced diet and practicing moderation is key, and starting your day with a full breakfast is important. MyPlate is the latest nutrition guide from the United States Department of Agriculture and is divided into four sections of approximately 30 percent grains, 30 percent vegetables, 20 percent fruits, and 20 percent protein, accompanied by a smaller circle representing dairy, such as milk or yogurt (20).

d. *Mindfulness*: This is the practice of maintaining a state of heightened or complete awareness of one's thoughts, emotions, or experiences without judgment in the given moment. For example, deep breathing for five minutes—inhaling for a count of four, holding for a count of two, and then exhaling for a count of four—enables one to focus and be mentally ready. When I go into a stressful situation, such as in the operating room or giving a talk in front of hundreds of people, I take three deep breaths to relax my body and focus my mind.

e. *Visualization or imagery:* This is the practice of visualizing the sequence of events to a task at hand which produces positive energy, confidence, and improves performance. For example, prior to any operation I do, I spend five minutes visualizing all the steps to the operation. This enables me to focus keenly with emphasis on what am I going to do if something goes wrong.

f. *Narrative writing or journaling:* This is the practice of writing down your positive and negative thoughts to separate you from these thoughts. Writing down each day could include three things that you are grateful for and why, three things that went well, and three things that did not go well and why. Further, it could be writing down "fail" on a piece of paper and then ripping it up prior to doing something you want to perform very well at, such as making a presentation, taking a test, or prior to participating in an athletic event.

g. *Setting and managing boundaries:* When you are on your way home, you can pick a time and area where you disconnect your work mind and focus on being present at home for your significant other, spouse, and children. Separating your work from your personal life is therapeutic and ensures you are living in the present.

YOUR "TACTICS"

My wife and I developed "TACTICS" to achieve a healthier, peaceful, and more purposeful life with optimum performance in mind, body, and spirit (see Image #11). We encourage you to practice your "TACTICS" daily to be your best:

- **T**ake time for yourself and lead a peaceful life
- **A**lways eat healthy, exercise, and sleep
- **C**ontinually self-improve and remain coachable
- **T**reasure family and friends

- **I** choose the day I have
- **C**ontrol disappointments and respond positively
- **S**mile and laugh

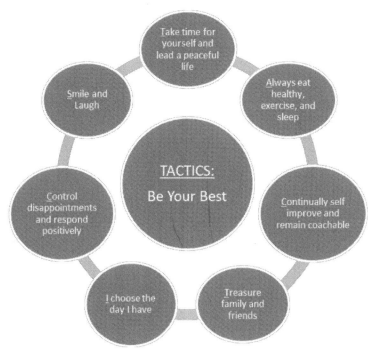

Image #11: TACTICS.

During my time at OSF HealthCare and Michigan State University, I have been involved with a variety of initiatives for others to learn to have better work-life balance. For example, at OSF, we developed a ministry-wide 45-minute seminar called "A conversation about work-life balance in a safe zone?" so physicians/staff have a safe place to listen and talk. At Michigan State University, we formed the Wellness & Patient Experience Committee to foster an environment that promotes healthy work-life balance, the continued physical and emotional development of our colleagues, role-modeling of professional and healthy behaviors, and compassionate recognition of unhealthy behaviors. From this committee, we decided on and implemented a survey instrument for providers to obtain a baseline work-life balance assessment, educated and raised awareness of signs and symptoms of burnout and resources available, and developed a peer support program for faculty and staff. Further, the employee assistant program provides an important resource at many organizations.

Conclusion

L ife is like a marathon. You need to pace yourself. You need to make plans and goals that are realistic. You need to ask for feedback to continually improve. You must be passionate about what you do. You need to think positive and eliminate negative thoughts. You need to feel the now and stay in the moment. You need not to have fear as fear stands for "face everything and respond" and not "forget everything and run." You need to celebrate your successes along the journey of life and not be too focused on climbing the ladder. Let the journey of life unfold. Be passionate and strike and ignite your work-life balance with your TACTICS!

Thank you for reading, and I hope I have provided you with a few tools to achieve a healthier, purposeful, and more peaceful life. It is important to reach out to a friend or colleague in time of need and listen as you can truly save a friend or colleague's life. Lastly, I like to share with you the following "train" poem by an unknown author that a colleague sent to me in time of need:

- Life is like a journey on a train . . . with its stations . . . with changes of routes . . . and with accidents!
- We board this train when we are born and our parents are the ones who get our ticket.
- We believe they will always travel on this train with us.
- However, at some station our parents will get off the train, leaving us alone on this journey.
- As time goes by, other passengers will board the train, many of whom will be significant—our siblings, friends, children, and even the love of our life.
- Many will get off during the journey and leave a permanent vacuum in our lives.
- Many will go so unnoticed that we won't even know when they vacated their seats and got off the train!
- This train ride will be full of joy, sorrow, fantasy, expectations, hellos, goodbyes, and farewells.
- A good journey is helping, loving, having a good relationship with all co-passengers. . . and making sure that we give our best to make their journey comfortable.
- The mystery of this fabulous journey is:
- We do not know at which station we ourselves are going to get off.
- So, we must live in the best way—adjust, forget, forgive and offer the best of what we have.
- It is important to do this because when the time comes for us to leave our seat . . . we should leave

behind beautiful memories for those who will continue to travel on the train of life.

- Thank you for being one of the important passengers on my train . . . don't know when my station will come . . . don't want to miss saying: "Thank you."

Acknowledgments

Over the past four years, I have had the opportunity to reflect on the many people that I have had the privilege to meet throughout my life who inspired me to help others achieve a healthier, peaceful, and purposeful life with optimum performance in mind, body, and spirit.

I would not be in the position I am in today without having loving relationships. My mother Jacqueline Proios, my father Louis Avellino, my stepfather Michael Proios, and my brother Greg Avellino, have always given me unconditional love, support, and guidance. Michael Proios has always treated me like his son, and I am so very thankful for his constant incredible wisdom. Further, my wife Jennifer, my daughter Ashleigh, my son Michael, and my dog Parker bring me much joy and are what I live for every day. Jennifer has been the very best wife and mother anyone could ask for. She has been my best friend, soulmate, and number one supporter. She loves being a mom and treasures her horse Levi and dog Parker. I continue to watch and guide Ashleigh and Michael to be their very best, and I'm in awe as they follow their passions along their life journey.

My neurosurgery mentors, Drs. Michel Kliot, H. Richard Winn, Richard G. Ellenbogen, Ted Roberts, Robert Goodkin, and Basil Harris have made me the neurosurgeon I am today. My many neurosurgery and orthopedic colleagues have also helped me provide the very best quality care, in specific Drs. Gavin Britz, Jim Schuster, Ben Carson, Jeff Ojemann, Jens Chapman, Sohail Mirza, Kit Song, Anand Veeravagu, Julian Lin, Casey Madura, and Michael Bercu; and Ann Biser, PA and Julie Deibel, APRN. My many administrative colleagues have guided me in being the very best leader, in specific Greta Torry, Johnese Spisso, Eileen Whalen, Steve Zieniewicz, Rod Hochman, Seth Ciabotti, and Sally Nogle.

I would like to thank my many friends for their guidance and always listening to me in time of need and having a way to bring me up when I am feeling down: Jake (my crab fishing captain) and Jenna Anderson, Adrian and Corinne Gomez, Chris (my ultra-running partner) and Mary Dierker, Eli and Rebecca Almo, Rob and Lynette Martin (Lynette has also provided valuable editorial assistance), Laurie and Dave Perry, Maribeth O'Connor, Jim and Katie Gaudino, Brad and Connie Fitterer, Jim Pignataro, Michael Capecci, Ken Horenstein, Anthony Manzi, Michael and Susan Guarnieri, Audrey Jones, Norman and Kristina Beauchamp, Laurie and Joe Thorp, Jane Powell, Ken and Jessica Berkovitz, Hallie Truswell (my longtime ultra-running coach), and John Rumpeltes (my long-time physical therapist).

Lastly, I want to thank the many patients and their families that have entrusted me with their care over the past 20 years, as I am continually inspired by their stories and their resilience.

References

Introduction

1. Portions of this section were adapted from: Avellino, Tony. "Is It Time to Bring Physician Burnout Out of the Shadows?" *Becker's Hospital Review*, March 30, 2017.

Part I: Listen (to discover your life's journey)

1. https://www.who.int/news-room/fact-sheets/detail/mental-health-strengthening-our-response (accessed November 17, 2019).
2. Truesdell, Jeff. "They Attempted Suicide and Survived: Here Are Their Stories." *People*, October 28, 2019, 65–66.
3. https://www.nami.org/nami/media/nami-media/infographics/generalmhfacts.pdf (accessed September 13, 2020).
4. Tikkanen, Roosa, and Melinda K. Abrams. "US Health Care from a Global Perspective, 2019: Higher Spending, Worse Outcomes." *The Commonwealth Fund, Data Brief*, January 2020, 1–19.

5. Lipson, Sarah Ketchen, Emily G. Lattie, and Daniel Eisenberg. "Increased Rates of Mental Health Service Utilization by U.S. College Students: 10-Year Population-Level Trends (2007-2017)." Psychiatric Services 70 (2019):60-63. DOI: 10.1176/appi.ps.201800332.

6. Yairi, Ehud and Nicoline Ambrose. "Epidemiology of Stuttering: 21st Century Advances." *Journal of Fluency Disorders* 38, Issue 2 (2013): 66–87. DOI:10.1016/j.jfludis.2012.11.002.

7. Azrin, NH and RG Nunn. "A Rapid Method of Eliminating Stuttering by a Regulated Breathing Approach." *Behaviour Research and Therapy* 12, Issue 4 (1974):279–286. PMID: 4447567.

Part II: Learn (from failures)

1. Frankel, Viktor. *Man's Search for Meaning: An Introduction to Logotherapy*. Boston, MA, Beacon Press, 2006. ISBN 978-0-8070-1427-1 (originally published in 1946).

2. Adapted from: Avellino, Tony and Debbie Kupfer. "Best Lesson: Faith Healing/Illness to Wellness." *GWISH Newsletter*, 2004.

3. Metcalf, Dan. *He Chose Joy!: The Story of Matthew Metcalf*. Bloomington, Indiana, WestBow Press, 2012.

4. Kohn, Linda T, Janet M. Corrigan, and Molla S. Donaldson, eds. *To Err Is Human: Building a Safer Health System*. Washington, D.C.: Institute of Medicine Committee on Quality of Health Care in America, National Academies Press, 2000. PMID: 25077248.

5. Portions of this section were adapted from: Avellino, Tony, Nick Mavar, Jr., and Dan Mattsen. "Other Voices— Health Care Leaders Can Learn from the Commercial Fishing Industry?" *The Anacortes American (Anacortes, Washington)*, November 20, 2013.

6. Avellino, Anthony Michael. *So You Want To Be A Doctor? A Guide For Those Interested In A Career In Medicine (Especially High School Students)*. New York, NY, Carlton Press, Inc., 1988. ISBN 0-8062-3116-5.

Part III: Heal (to achieve a healthier and more purposeful life)

1. Bezdek, Kylie Garber, and Eva H. Telzer. "Have No Fear, the Brain Is Here! How Your Brain Responds to Stress." *Frontiers for Young Minds* 5, Article 71 (2017):1–8. DOI: 10.3389/frym.2017.00071.

2. Lutz, Jacqueline, Uwe Herwig, Sarah Opialla, Anna Hittmeyer, Lutz Jäncke, Michael Rufer, Martin Grosse Holtforth, and Annette B. Brühl. "Mindfulness and Emotion Regulation—an fMRI Study." *Social Cognitive and Affective Neuroscience* 9, Issue 6 (2014):776–785.

3. Adapted from Dr. David Hanscom, orthopaedic surgeon; David Elaimy, golf teacher and coach; and Gallwey, W. Timothy. *The Inner Game of Work: Focus, Learning, Pleasure, and Mobility in the Workplace*. New York, Random House Trade Paperbacks, 2001. ISBN-10: 9780375758171.

4. McDonald, Judy, Terry Orlick, and Merv Letts. "Mental Readiness in Surgeons and Its Links to Performance Excellence in Surgery." *Journal of Pediatric Orthopedics* 15 (1995):691–697. PMID: 7593587.

5. Coyle, Daniel. *The Talent Code*. New York, New York, Bantam Book, 2009.

6. Gladwell, Malcom. *Outliers*. New York, New York, Little, Brown and Company, 2008.

7. Maslach, Christina, and Susan E. Jackson. "The Measurement of Experienced Burnout." *Journal of Occupational Behavior* 2 (1981):99–113.

8. Rene A. Spitz (1945) "Hospitalism: An Inquiry into the Genesis of Psychiatric Conditions in Early Childhood." *The Psychoanalytic Study of the Child* (1945):53–74. DOI: 10.1080/00797308.1945.11823126.

9. Nerem, Robert M., Murina J. Levesque, and J. Fredrick Cornhill. "Social Environment as a Factor in Diet-induced Atherosclerosis." *Science* 208 (1980):1475–1476. PMID: 7384790.

10. Becher, Rabbi Mordechai. *Gateway to Judaism*. Brooklyn, New York, Shaar Press, 2005.

11. Studer, Quint and George Ford. *Healing Physician Burnout*. Pensacola, Florida, Fire Starter Publishing, 2015.

12. Hartman, Micah, Anne B. Martin, Joseph Benson, Aaron Catlin, and the National Health Expenditure Accounts Team. "National Health Care Spending in 2018: Growth Driven by Accelerations in Medicare and Private Insurance Spending." *Health Affairs* 39, No. 1 (2020):8–17. DOI: 10.1377/hlthaff.2019.01451.

13. Shanafelt, Tait D., Colin P. West, Christine Sinsky, Mickey Trockel, Michael Tutty, Daniel V. Satele, Lindsey E. Carlasare, and Lotte N. Dyrbye. "Changes in Burnout and

Satisfaction with Work-Life Integration in Physicians and the General US Working Population between 2011 and 2017." *Mayo Clinic Proceedings* 94 (2019):1681–1694.

14. Shanafelt, Tait D., Omar Hasan, Lotte N. Dyrbye, Christine Sinsky, Daniel Satele, Jeff Sloan, and Colin P. West. "Changes in Burnout and Satisfaction with Work-Life Balance in Physicians and the General US Working Population between 2011 and 2014." *Mayo Clinic Proceedings* 90 (2015):1600–1613.

15. Weber, David Ollier. "Battling Physician Burnout, Part 1: Too Many Doctors Are Struggling with Stress, and Too Few Organizations Are Helping Them." *Hospitals & Health Networks—AHA Publication*, June 25, 2013. https://www.hhnmag.com/articles/5664-battling-physician-burnout-part-1.

16. Han, Shasha, Tait D. Shanafelt, Christine A. Sinsky, Karim M. Awad, Liselotte N. Dyrbye, Lynne C. Fiscus, Mickey Trockel, and Joel Goh. "Estimating the Attributable Cost of Physician Burnout in the United States." *Annals of Internal Medicine* 170 (2019):784–790. DOI: 10.7326/M18-1422.

17. Loehr, Jim and Tony Schwartz. "The Making of a Corporate Athlete." *Harvard Business Review*, January 2001 Issue.

18. Chaput, Jean-Philippe, Caroline Dutil, and Hugues Sampasa-Kanyinga. "Sleeping Hours: What Is the Ideal Number and How Does Age Impact This?" *Nature and Science of Sleep* 10 (2018):421–430. PMID: 30568521.

19. For "Physical Activity Guidelines for Americans" see: https://www.hhs.gov/fitness/be-active/physical-activity-guidelines-for-americans/index.html.
20. For "Dietary Guidelines for Americans" see: a) https://foh.psc.gov/calendar/nutrition.html, b) https://www.choosemyplate.gov/, and c) https://www.dietaryguidelines.gov/current-dietary-guidelines/2015-2020-dietary-guidelines.

Index

Page numbers followed by "*f*" refer to figures.

About the Author

Anthony M. Avellino is a highly regarded pediatric neurosurgeon, experienced healthcare administrator, and endurance ultra-runner who has battled with depression, obsessive-compulsive tendencies, suicide, and stuttering as long as he can remember. In October 2019 and January 2021, Avellino was fortunate to be a deckhand on the F/V *Saga*, a commercial crab fishing boat profiled on the Discovery show *Deadliest Catch*. He built his career caring for young people and their families, including a deliberate focus on creating support systems that emphasize performance, health, wellness, and safety. He started his pediatric neurosurgery career at Johns Hopkins University Hospital, where he was privileged to be Dr. Ben Carson's partner. He is presently the Michigan State University assistant vice president for health sciences, chief clinical and medical officer, and interim director of athletic medicine. Prior to joining MSU in 2018, he served as chief executive officer for OSF HealthCare Illinois Neurological

Institute from 2014 to 2018. Under his leadership, the Illinois Neurological Institute rankings, net revenue, contribution margin, outpatient visits, and hospital encounters significantly increased. In 2009, he was the first director of the UW Medicine Neurosciences Institute for the University of Washington Medicine and was also appointed chief of neurological surgery at the University of Washington Medical Center in 2011. He is a former NCAA student-athlete at Cornell University. He completed his medical education at Columbia University, his neurosurgery residency at the University of Washington, including a year as a specialist registrar at Atkinson Morley's Hospital in Wimbledon, England, and a pediatric neurosurgery fellowship at Seattle Children's Hospital.

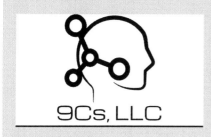

9Cs, LLC, Consulting Services

Engagement Services

Do you want to bring joy back into your life and achieve life-long wellness, success, and work-life balance?

Learn from a brain surgeon how to optimize your performance in mind, body, and spirit!

I founded 9Cs, a consulting service, which provides motivational talks, interactive workshops, and tools, to empower one to begin their journey to lead a healthier, peaceful, and purposeful life through my listen-learn-heal approach. I will provide three tools to help one begin their journey: Hills of Life, Life Balance Sheet, and TACTICS.

I would welcome the opportunity to work with your team. To learn more, please contact me at findingpurpose37@gmail.com.

Sincerely,
Anthony M. Avellino, MD, MBA
Founder of 9Cs, LLC

Mission, Vision, Values

Mission: To help one achieve their optimum performance in wellness and safety goals to lead a healthier, peaceful, and purposeful life through listening, learning, and healing.

Vision: To be recognized as the most value-added wellness and safety consultants at the national and international levels.

Values: We believe in providing the ideal environment for your organization to achieve success through the values of compassion, vulnerability, accountability, continuous improvement, and transformational change.

Areas of Focus

1. *Performance and Wellness (Performance = Skill – Interference)*
   a. To optimize one's performance in mind, body, and spirit
   b. To achieve life-long wellness, success, and work-life balance
   c. To raise awareness of mental health and addiction

2. *Safety Learning ("healthcare vs commercial fishing")*
   a. Safety is freedom

- How to translate "my life is at risk?"
  - ° HIV, COVID-19 pandemic
- Goals:
  - ° How to prevent mishaps?
  - ° "What If" scenarios?
  - ° How to create a safer and compliant system or process?
  - ° What went wrong and what we are doing to fix it in what timeline?
- Strategy:
  - ° Design
  - ° Construction
  - ° Maintenance
  - ° Allocation of resources
  - ° Training
  - ° Developing standard policies/procedures (e.g., checklists)
b. Teamwork, Communication, and Leadership Training

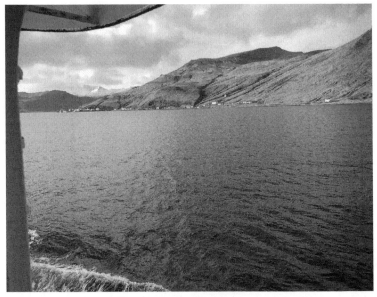

Dutch Harbor, Alaska 2019 (Photo by author).

Made in United States
Orlando, FL
24 January 2022

13977956R00067